Diseases of Horses - The Respiratory Organs and the Alimentary Canal

With Information on Diagnosis and Treatment

By

A H Baker

British Library Cataloguing-in-Publication Data
A catalogue record for this book is available from the
British Library

Horses – Breeding and Anatomy

The horse (*Equus ferus caballus*) is one of two extant subspecies of *Equus ferus*. It is an odd-toed ungulate mammal belonging to the taxonomic family 'Equidae'. The horse has evolved over the past 45 to 55 million years from a small multi-toed creature into the large, single-toed animal of today. Humans began to domesticate horses around 4000 BC, and their domestication is believed to have been widespread by 3000 BC. We, as humans have interacted with horses in a multitude of ways throughout history – from sport competitions and non-competitive recreational pursuits, to working activities such as police work, agriculture, entertainment and therapy. Horses have also been used in warfare, from which a wide variety of riding and driving techniques developed, using many different styles of equipment and methods of control. With this range of uses in mind, there is an equally extensive, specialized vocabulary used to describe equine-related concepts, covering everything from anatomy to life stages, size, colours, markings, breeds, locomotion, and behaviour. Horse anatomy is a fascinating topic, and in the course of this introduction, the basics will be discussed.

To start; the horse skeleton averages 250 bones. A significant difference between the horse skeleton and that of a human is the lack of a collarbone—the horse's forelimbs are attached to the spinal column by a powerful set of muscles, tendons, and ligaments that attach the shoulder blade to the torso. The horse's legs and hooves are also unique structures. Their leg bones are proportioned differently from those of a human. For example, the body part that is called a horse's 'knee' is actually made up of the carpal bones that correspond to the human wrist. Similarly, the hock contains bones equivalent to those in the human ankle and heel. A horse also has no muscles in its legs below the knees and hocks, only skin, hair, bone, tendons, ligaments, cartilage, and the assorted specialized tissues that make up the hoof.

The hoof is one of the most important to study, and easily damaged parts of a horse. The critical importance of the feet and legs is summed up by the traditional adage, 'no foot, no horse.' The exterior hoof wall and horn of the sole is made of essentially the same material as a human fingernail. The end result is that a horse, weighing on average 500 kilograms (1,100 lb), travels on the same bones as would a human on tiptoe. For the protection of the hoof under certain conditions, some horses have horseshoes placed on their feet by a professional farrier. The hoof continually grows, and in most domesticated horses needs to be trimmed (and horseshoes reset, if used) every five to eight weeks, though the hooves of horses in the wild wear down and regrow at a rate suitable for their terrain.

One of the most important aspects of equine care is farriery. Farriers have largely replaced blacksmiths (after this specialism largely became redundant after the industrial revolution), and are highly skilled in both metalwork and horse anatomy. Historically, the jobs of farrier and blacksmith were practically synonymous, shown by the etymology of the word: farrier comes from Middle French *ferrier* (blacksmith), and from the Latin word *ferrum* (iron). Modern day farriers usually specialize in horseshoeing though, focusing their time and effort on the care of the horse's hoof, including trimming and balancing of the hoof, as well as the placing of the shoes. Additional tasks for the farrier include dealing with injured or diseased hooves and application of special shoes for racing, training or 'cosmetic' purposes. In countries such as the United Kingdom, it is illegal for people other than registered farriers to call themselves a farrier or to carry out any farriery work, the primary aim being 'to prevent and avoid suffering by and cruelty to horses arising from the shoeing of horses by unskilled persons.' This is not the case in all countries however, where horse protection is severely lacking.

The terrain horses originally inhabited is crucial to understanding their anatomy; horses are naturally grazing creatures. In an adult horse, there are 12 incisors at the front of the mouth, adapted to biting off the grass or other vegetation, with 24 teeth adapted for chewing. Stallions and geldings have four additional teeth just behind the incisors, a type of canine teeth called 'tushes.' Some horses, both male and female, will also develop one to four very small vestigial teeth in front of the molars, known as 'wolf' teeth, which are generally removed because they can interfere with the bit. As horses are herbivores, their grazing nature has resulted in a digestive system adapted to steady consumption of grasses. Therefore, compared to humans, they have a relatively small stomach but very long intestines to facilitate a steady flow of nutrients. Interestingly, horses are unable to vomit – so digestion problems can arise quickly, causing colic, a leading killer.

Horse breeds are loosely divided into three categories based on general temperament: spirited 'hot bloods' with speed and endurance; 'cold bloods', such as draft horses and some ponies, suitable for slow, heavy work; and 'warm bloods', developed from crosses between hot bloods and cold bloods, often focusing on creating breeds for specific riding purposes, particularly in Europe. There are more than 300 breeds of horse in the world today, developed for many different uses. The concept of purebred bloodstock and a controlled, written breed registry has become particularly significant; sometimes inaccurately described as 'thoroughbreds'. Thoroughbred is a specific breed of horse, while a 'purebred' is a horse (or any other animal) with a defined pedigree recognized by a breed registry. An early example of people who practiced selective horse breeding were the Bedouin, who had a reputation for careful practices, keeping extensive pedigrees of their Arabian horses and placing great value upon pure bloodlines. In the fourteenth century, Carthusian monks of southern Spain kept meticulous pedigrees of bloodstock lineages still found today in the Andalusian horse.

We hope the reader enjoys this book, and is encouraged to explore the world of horse breeding and anatomy for themselves.

I. TUMOR IN THE FALSE NOSTRIL.——II. POLYPUS.——III. CATARRH.——IV. NASAL GLEET.——V. LARYNGITIS, ROARING AND WHISTLING.——VI. QUINSY.——VII. BRONCHITIS.——VIII. PNEUMONIA.——IX. HEAVES.——X. CONGESTION OF THE LUNGS.——XI. PLEURISY.——XII. HYDROTHORAX.——XIII. CHRONIC COUGH.

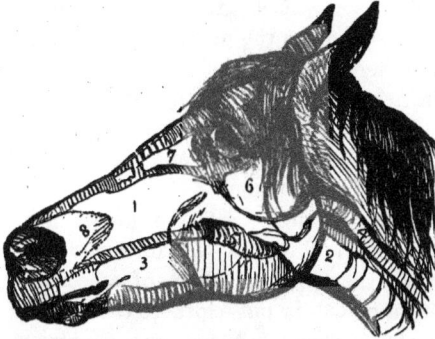

DIAGRAM SHOWING RESPIRATORY ORGANS IN THE HEAD OF A HORSE.

1.—The nostril leading direct to 2.—The larynx, situated at the commencement of the windpipe. 3.—The tongue. 4.—The œsophagus or gullet. 5.—The soft palate, which lies upon the tongue and affords a resting-place whereon reposes the epiglottis, or the guardian cartilage to the entrance of the larynx (2). 6.—The guttural pouches, or large membranous and open sacs, containing nothing but atmospheric air. 7.—Nasal or frontal sinuses. 8.—The false nostril.

I. Tumor in the False Nostril.

The **false nostril** is the small pouch or *cul de sac* on the outer side of the lower edge of each nostril. Tumors are liable to form in these, and partake more of the nature of abscesses, in that they are filled with pus of a cheesy consistency, but are tumors in that they form slowly and do not point and break like an abscess. They are usually about the size of a hen's egg; they are not sore, but cause more or less wheezing in the breathing on account of the diminished capacity of the air passage.

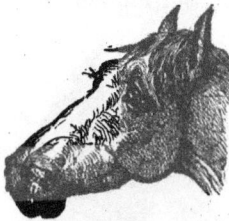

FACE OF HORSE.

Showing appearance of muzzle when there is a tumor in the false nostril.

How to know it.—A small swelling will be apparent on the outside, but the main dependence is to be placed upon the examination of the nostril, when it will be found to be nearly closed by the tumor in the false nostril.

What to do.--It can be opened without the slightest danger. Insert the knife inside the nostril and make a free opening and evacuate the pus. Inject lotion No. 6, twice a day. It is not likely to recur.

II. Polypus.

This is a tumor-like excrescence growing in the nostril. It may form in any part of the passage from the muzzle to the throat. It is usually a fleshy bulb, on a pedestal or neck. It varies in size from a cherry to a man's fist.

How to know it.—The breathing is obstructed, to a certain extent, and, upon examination, the polypus is found.

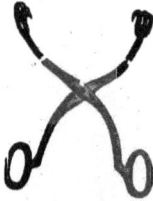

What to do.—Cast the horse, and catch firm hold of it with the forceps for the pur pose, then pass the chain of an *ecraseur* over it, and cut it out close to the surface from which it grows. A fine copper wire may be used, if the *ecraseur* cannot be had; pass the wire over the polypus and twist it off. There will not be hemorrhage to do any harm. The polypus may grow again, but it is not very likely to.

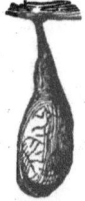

FORCEPS.

For grasping the polypus for removal.

POLYPUS.

Hanging from the upper part of the nostril.

III. Catarrh.

Under this name are included acute catarrh and the common cold when it is confined to the nose. It is simple in itself, but all inflammations of the upper air-passages are liable to run down into the lungs and cause bronchitis and pneumonia, which are always serious. Catarrh is inflammation of the mucous membrane of the nostrils, and often extends to the sinuses of the head, especially the frontal sinuses situated between the eyes.

Causes.—Exposure to cold winds, rain and snow storms, cold nights, etc.

How to know it.—There is always a discharge from one or both nostrils. The discharge is thin watery mucous at first, and turns to muco-purulent in the course of a couple of days; and then to purulent, if not properly treated. The muco-purulent is white and frothy; the purulent is yellow, and has an offensive

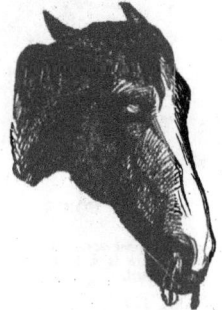

A HORSE'S HEAD WITH COLD.

2

odor. In bad cases, there is considerable fever, loss of appetite, and

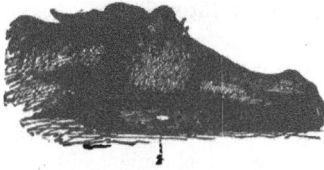

LYMPHATIC GLAND OF THROAT SWOLLEN.

1—The enlarged lymphatic within the jaw.

redness of the eyes. If neglected, and nature is not vigorous enough to throw it off, it becomes chronic, and is known as nasal gleet. Sometimes the lymphatic gland, under the lower jaw, enlarges.

What to do.—Remove the cause; if exposed to cold storms, shelter the animal, put on a blanket if necessary, feed on soft feed, give a teaspoonful of saltpetre in a bran mash night and morning. If that does not perform the work satisfactorily, give the fever mixture, No. 4. If there is much fever and loss of appetite, give No. 18. In all bad cases, give rest till the horse is better. If the attack is prolonged to a week or more, during convalesence, give the tonic No. 22, and syringe the nostrils out, two or three times a day, with the following lotion:

No. 39.

2 Drachms carbolic acid,
1 Pint of water,
Mix.

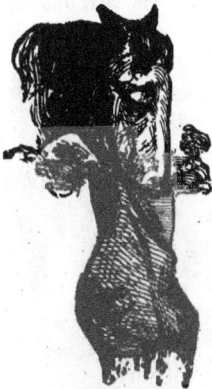

NOSE BAG.
For steaming horse with cold.

Apply the blister No. 41 to the throat, letting it go well up towards the ears. If the skin is not mildly blistered with one application, repeat it after twenty-four hours; then grease it once a day with fresh lard. When the discharge does not come freely, it can be helped by steaming the head in a bag of hot bran.

IV. Nasal Gleet.

This is the name given to chronic catarrh, and is always complicated by extension of the disease to the sinuses of the

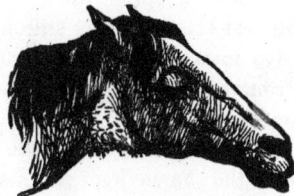

A HORSE WITH THE THROAT BLISTERED.

head, often causing the bone over the one affected to bulge out, as if swollen.

Causes.—Neglected or obstinate catarrh, that will not yield to treatment with an ordinary amount of perseverance, are the only causes. The sinuses of the head are all in communication with each other by tubes and passages. When inflammation extends to them, the swelling of the mucous membrane closes these passages, and confines the pus with suffi-

3

cient force to cause the bones to bulge out, but there will be a constant flow of pus from the nostril, sufficient being forced through the passage by the pressure to keep up the discharge.

How to know it.—The general health is not in the least affected, except, perhaps, in long standing cases. There is a continual flow of thick, offensive, yellowish matter that will usually sink in water. One nostril usually runs more than the other, and oftentimes the chronic trouble is entirely confined to one side. The face between the eyes will be found to be full, giving a dull, solid sound when tapped on each side of the median line running down the centre of the face. In long standing, bad cases the bone of the face, referred to above, will be bulged out, and great pain evinced when tapped.

Pus is, naturally, the blandest secretion of the body; but being confined, it corrupts, and then smells abominably. The facial sinuses formed in nasal gleet, open to the nostrils on either side by two comparatively small flaps, slits or valves. These are their only means of communication with the external atmosphere; and through these valves all the pus must flow. It is not surprising that such structures occasionally become clogged, till the accumulated secretion, or the increased breathing, or the position of the head, obliges the passage to give way.

What to do.—If the sinus is full, there is no cure for it without the operation of trephining to remove a portion of the bone, to evacuate the sinus, and give local treatment; but if there is no bulging of the bone, it may be cured by syringing out the nostril with warm water to clean it, then injecting a little of lotion No. 39 with a long-nozzled syringe, using considerable force to cause a spray when it strikes the back of the nose. Repeat this, morning and night, for a month or so, and give internally, No. 34. The operation of trephining the frontal sinus, will be found described in the chapter on operations.

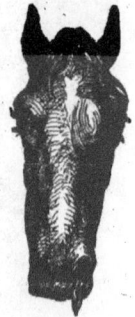

NASAL GLEET. Horse affected with nasal gleet and bulging of the frontal sinus.

All treatment, except the operation, may be continued and the horse kept at his work, unless he is laid up on account of the appearance of the nostril, as it looks very bad to drive a horse with a chronic discharge from the nose.

V. Laryngitis, Roaring and Whistling.

This is what is ordinarily known as sore throat. The inflammation lies in the lining of the larynx—that is, the cartilaginous box in the throat, which is the upper end of the windpipe or *trachea* containing the vocal cords, and is the seat of roaring.

Causes.—Exposure to cold winds and storms, standing in drafts when warm, neglect when coming in when warm from work, and extension of catarrh from the nose. The cause of roaring is chronic inflammation of the mucous membrane lining the larynx, diminishing the air passage so that when he is unable to get sufficient air, and forcing it through the small passage, makes the noise.

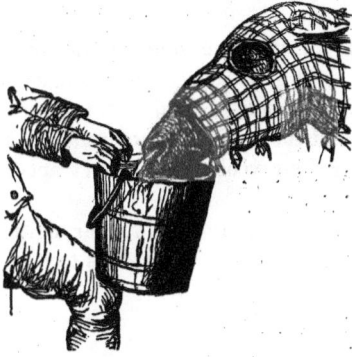

EFFECT OF LARYNGITIS.

A horse trying to drink, the water returning by the nose.

How to know it.—The throat is usually swollen on the outside, but sometimes only on the inside, and is tender upon pressure; the nose is protruded; he has great difficulty in swallowing, and often, when drinking, the water will come back through the nose nearly as fast as it goes into the mouth, and what is swallowed is forced down with an effort. There is usually a short, painful, subdued cough, dry at first, but getting more moist after a couple of days.

What to do.—Clothe warmly; shelter from cold storms and drafts; rub mustard paste well into the throat on each side, well up towards the ears; feed on soft mashes, boiled oats, etc., and set a pail of water in the manger for him to play in to cool the throat and mouth. Give internally fever mixture No. 4, every two hours till the fever is reduced and the pulse lowered; then drop off to three or four times a day. If the swelling in the throat does not yield to the above treatment, apply a soft, hot linseed poultice to it, and change it once a day for a fresh one. The loss of appetite, or rather inability to eat, will soon disappear and recovery will be rapid.

In case of roaring, apply a smart blister of cantharides, No. 9, to the throat, and after three weeks repeat it. Inject a tablespoonful of the mixture No. 35, three times a day well back into the throat, and let the horse run at grass or feed on very soft food.

Bad, long standing cases of roaring are incurable. Whistling is similar to roaring, except in the noise produced; it is subject to the same causes and treatment.

Roaring and whistling are sometimes, but very rarely, the effect of paralysis of the nerves of the larynx, letting one or more of the cartilages drop into the box to a certain extent, and thereby diminishing the caliber of the air passage. Sometimes a small portion of the cartilage doing the damage can be removed, but it requires the skill of a qualified veterinary surgeon.

5

VI. Quinsy.

Causes.—Sometimes the inflammation in the throat in laryngitis is so great and deep seated that abscesses form in the throat, producing quinsy. It is caused by the same agents as laryngitis, and is always more prolonged in duration than simple sore throat.

How to know it.—It may start with all the symptoms of laryngitis but will not yield to treatment at first. The throat gets sorer and sorer from day to day, till suddenly the abscess bursts, and a tremendous flow of pus comes from the nostril, and the animal will be relieved at once. Quinsy lasts from one to three or four weeks, and is very apt to be followed by roaring or whistling.

What to do.—Apply the same treatment as prescribed for laryngitis. Continue the linseed poultices right through; apply them so as to cover the throat nearly to the ears, and keep them quite soft.

VII. Bronchitis.

The bronchial tubes are the two branches of the trachea or wind pipe; they lead to the lungs. Inflammation of these branches, and also of the lining of the tubes as **they ramify** through the lungs, is known as bronchitis.

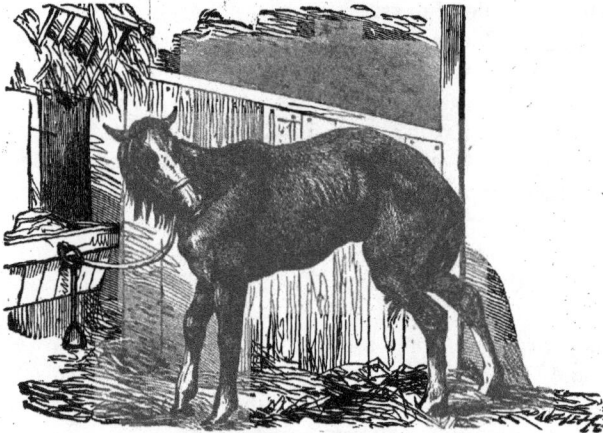

A FIT SUBJECT FOR FOUNDER OR BRONCHITIS.

Causes.—The same exposures that cause catarrh and sore throat are prolific agents in producing this disease. And there is a very great tendency in the horse to inflammations of the upper air passages which run down upon the lungs, so much so that many cases of catarrh and laryngitis terminate in bronchitis **and pneumonia.**

6

How to know it.—It is always ushered in with a shivering fit, but this fit is seldom seen, and if seen is thought nothing of by most people; the chill passes off and the reaction brings fever; the pulse runs up to fifty or sixty, is soft, full and bounding; temperature soon runs up to 102 ° or 103 ° F.; the breathing is hurried and the nostrils are distended. If pressure is applied to the chest just above the breast bone. pain will be evinced and a cough provoked, which is soft, deep and subdued, great pain being manifested while coughing; the horse is loth to move; if the ear is placed to the nostril a grunt will be heard with each breath; and if the ear is placed in front of the chest a thick, unnatural sound will be heard; the ears and legs are usually cold; the appetite is indifferent. All of these symptoms will be noticed in the course of ten or twelve hours. In the next twenty-four hours the pulse may run up to 70, and the temperature to 104.° or 105 ° ; the pulse will be soft and full; the cough will increase and the thick, heavy sound when the ear is applied to

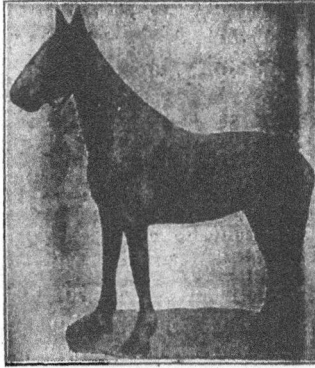

HORSE WITH BRONCHITIS.

the breast will have run into a harsh, grating sound; the horse persistently stands; drinks considerable water, and the appetite will be lost in most cases; the mouth will be hot to the finger placed under the tongue; the breath is hot as it comes from the nostrils, and the urine is scanty and high colored. The horse may die from continuation of the inflammation and extension of it to the lungs proper, or may drown in the mucus that is secreted in the passages forming the next stage following the dry one; in this last a rattling bubbling sound is heard when the ear is applied to the chest above the breast bone, by the air rushing through the mucus.

Convalescence will be noticed by a diminution of the mucous rattle; falling of the pulse and temperature; return of the appetite; and a generally relieved appearance; ability to lie down and rest quietly, and the frequency of the breathing lessened.

7

What to do.—If seen during the chill, give two ounces of whiskey in a little water and follow it with No. 4, for the next twelve hours; then, if better, continue the same at longer intervals, but if worse, change it to the following:

No. 40.
1 ½ Ounce sweet spirits of nitre,
1 Drachm tincture of aconite root,
2 Drachms fluid extract belladonna,
1 Ounce tincture of gentian,
1 Ounce powdered saltpetre,
1 Ounce powdered sal ammoniæ,
Water to make one pint,
Mix.

Give a wine-glassful every two nours till the horse is better, then drop off to three or four times a day. Set a bucket of water in his manger. Give scalded oats to eat; if he won't eat them try him with other things

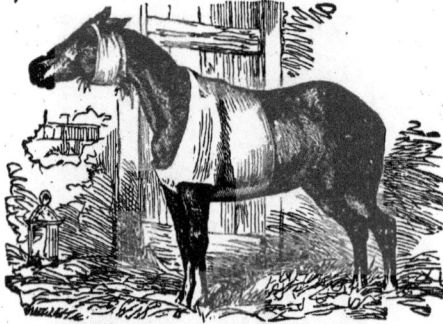

A HORSE DRESSED FOR BRONCHITIS.

—a couple of ears of corn three or four times a day, carrots, apples, good hay, etc. Rub a little of the following liniment well into the sides over the lungs, and on the chest once a day till it is well blistered:

No. 41.
2 Ounces liquor ammonia,
2 Ounces spirits turpentine,
2 Ounces linseed oil,
Mix and shake.

When the blistering has been carried far enough, rub a little fresh lard well into the hair once a day to take out the scabs without pulling out the hair. If the skin comes off anywhere from the blister, apply No. 24 to the spot three times a day.

Give plenty of pure air to breathe, but avoid drafts and dampness; see that the drainage is good. Remove him from the other horses if possible, on account of the vitiated air he would have to breathe in the stable with them.

When convalescence is well established and there is much weakness, change the medicine to No. 18, but do not give it as often as every two hours, unless there is still a good deal of fever; three times a day is often enough in most cases.

When the fever is all gone, change the medicine to No. 35, if the appetite is poor, but if it is good, give No. 34 in the feed. Give gentle exercise when well enough to bear it. The horse should be well clothed, and the legs bandaged. Bring him back to his feed and work gradually. While wearing the bandages they should be removed morning and night, and the legs well rubbed and the bandages replaced.

VIII. Pneumonia.

This is inflammation of the lung tissue; oftentimes the right lung only is affected. Pneumonia is rather rare, at least it is far less common than bronchitis, and sometimes the two diseases are combined in the form of broncho-pneumonia. It may be either sporadic or infectious. In the latter case it is seen as a complication of influenza, and has typhoid symptoms, and is occasionally enzoötic, or may be epizoötic.

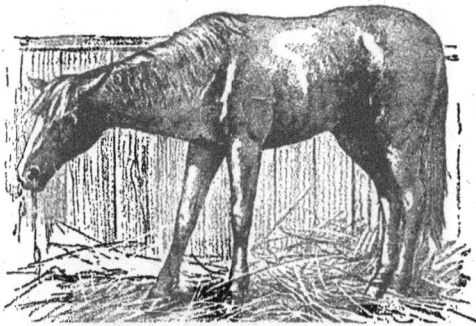

HORSE WITH CHEST AILMENT.
Front feet spread.   Strong running of the nose after coughing.

Causes.—The same as for other acute affections of the air passages, except when existing as a complication of influenza, then it is due to a micro-organism (the pneumococcus). The sporadic form will usually recover if given a fair chance, but the infectious is frequently fatal.

How to know it.—The first stage is the shivering fit and sanguineous congestion, in which there is a rush of blood to the lungs; high fever follows the chill, the pulse runs up to sixty to eighty, and is soft and weak; the temperature is likely to run up to 105° to 107° Fahr. The breath is hot, and breathing labored and fast—respirations running up to twenty-five to thirty-five per minute; the ear being applied to the sides, the grating sound indicative of inflammation is heard; there is no cough; ears and legs are cold; the body heat is great, and the urine scanty and high colored.

The second stage is that of hepatization, in which the lungs become solid, like liver; no sound is heard at all by the ear when applied to the side, and, when tapped, it sounds solid like a barrel when full of water—the natural when tapped being resonant, like a drum. The lower part of the lung being usually most affected, the breathing is floated upward, as it were, and becomes shallow; the breath becomes cold in consequence; the nostrils flap, and the horse thrusts his nose through the windows or doors of the stable in search of more air; the flanks heave; the ribs are worked violently in and out; the legs spread to stand in a braced position; the strength becomes exhausted, and the system suffocates for want of oxygen, and the animal usually dies in this stage.

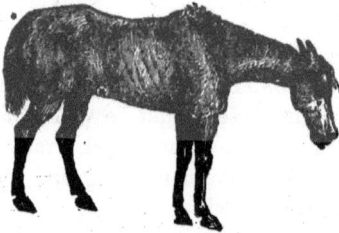

HORSE WITH PNEUMONIA.
The appearance of a horse in the early stage of pneumonia.

If he lives through this stage, the third stage begins—that of absorption; in favorable cases this goes on to so great an extent that recovery is complete. Unfavorable cases fail to absorb the liver-like condition of the lung, and suppuration sets in; the whole diseased portion may turn to pus, and be thrown up through the nose, where it has a grayish, lumpy appearance. This is the fourth stage, and is always fatal; the discharge is extremely offensive, attracting hosts of flies and rendering a whole stable unfit for other horses to remain in.

In this, as in bronchitis, the horse never lies down till he is very much better, or nearly well.

In infectious pneumonia, in addition to the above symptoms, there will be marked yellowness of the mucous membranes, more rapidly developing weakness than in the sporadic form, and occasionally diarrhœa and other symptoms of influenza.

What to do.—The same treatment prescribed for bronchitis will apply to this, and, in addition, during recovery, if weakness is great, give malt ale in pint drenches three times a day. If

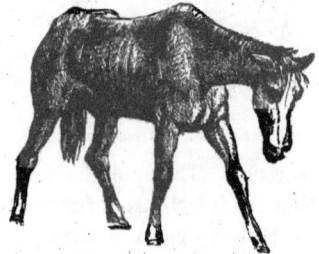

THE POSITION ASSUMED BY THE HORSE DURING AN ATTACK OF PNEUMONIA.

there is no appetite, put the ale in with oatmeal gruel, and give them as a drench together. Clothe him warmly, and give plenty of fresh air to breathe, but avoid a draft. It is a good plan, when feasible, to isolate him from all other horses, particularly in the infectious form.

10

If the fever remains above 104° F. longer than three days give the follow،
ing mixture:

> No. 91. ½ Ounce sulphate of quinine,
> 1 Pint of whisky,
> ½ Pint of water.
> Mix.

Give a wineglassful every two to four hours, alternating with the following mixture:

> No. 92. 1 Ounce tincture of nux vomica,
> 1 Ounce tincture of gentian,
> Water to make one pint.
> Mix.

Give a wineglassful every two to four hours.

Keep the stable clean and sprinkle chloride of lime around it freely once
a day. Give no exercise till convalescence is well established.

IX. Heaves.

The lungs are made up of an innumerable quantity of small air cells,
and the lung tissue is capable, to a great extent, of expelling the air from
it, and drawing more in by virtue of the elasticity and contractility it
possesses. Sometimes many of these cells become ruptured into one large
cell, which destroys the contractility of that portion of the lung, in which
case the diaphragm, ribs and abdominal muscles are brought into use to
expel the air, giving rise to the second spasmodic, twitching effort seen
in the flanks. This condition constitutes heaves, also known as broken
wind.

Causes.—The most common cause is driving too fast, and keeping it up
too long when the horse is not in condition—either having his stomach too
full and not giving the lungs room, or the lungs themselves are weak
from very light work, or entire disuse. Horses fed entirely on dusty
Timothy hay, are more subject to it than those fed on prairie hay. A
horse is more likely to get the heaves when driven fast against the wind
than with it; the lungs get very full of air, immensely distended by the
extra amount taken in, and if kept at that kind of work any length of
time, the lung tissue gives way, and a rupture is the consquence.

How to know it.—Instead of the regular, easy breathing noticed in the
flanks, there is a second effort made by the jerking of the muscles of the
flank. When the ear is placed against the side over the lung, a whistling,
wheezing sound is usually heard. When once begun it is very apt to
increase, and often renders the horse useless.

What to do.—It is incurable, but it can be alleviated by careful feed،
ing, giving as condensed food as possible, with a view of getting the
greatest amount of nourishment in the smallest compass. Wet everything

he eats, to lay the dust. Give the following mixture twice a day in soft feed:

No. 42. 2 Ounces powdered lobelia seed.
2 Ounces linseed meal,
Mix.

Divide into eight doses; give one night and morning. When they are gone, wait a week and repeat it. Avoid giving too much, as it is apt to weaken the kidneys. Always drive a horse slowly that has the heaves.

X. Congestion of the Lungs.

Congestion, is always a precursor of inflammation of the lungs, but it sometimes comes on in such a way, as to need separate consideration. The pathology of it is turgescence of the lung tissue by stagnation of the capillary blood vessels and arterioles. Under favorable circumstances it improves, and total recovery is the result, but in bad cases it is very apt to run on to inflammation of the lung tissue, and a case of pneumonia is the result.

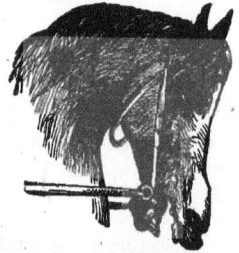

BAD POSITION.

For head of horse affected with heaves; for it aggravates the difficult breathing.

Causes.—Over exertion when not in condition to take it; the system is fat; the blood is rich and fat; the lung tissue is weak from want of use during longer or shorter periods of idleness. When in this condition, the horse is taken out, perhaps, once a week, and the driver thinks because he has had so long a rest, he ought to be able to go faster than if he were out every day, and sends him through to beat the crowd. Congestion of the lungs is quite frequently the result. This is oftener seen in the old country among the hunters, but is not infrequent in this country among the gentlemen's road horses. From the contraction of the muscular tissue, the blood is thrown inwardly to the lungs, liver and spleen; the lung tissue becomes fatigued, and the small blood vessels surcharged with blood to such an extent as to interfere with the circulation.

How to know it.—The horse suddenly stops, all out of breath; nostrils distended; the countenance has a look of anxiety upon it; he looks around as if in search for more air; paws the ground in his endeavor to breathe, and acts generally as though suffocation were near.

What to do.—Let him stop; turn his head towards the wind; loosen all harness that interferes with the free expansion of the chest and passage of air to the chest; let down the check rein; loosen the throat lash; remove the collar or breast plate and girth; and a small stab of the knife in the roof of the mouth to draw a little blood may assist in restoring the circulation. As soon as he is sufficiently recovered, take him home quietly

12

and place him in a comfortable loose box; give him a sponge bath with alcohol and plenty of friction from head to foot; also cold water to drink in small quantities, and give recipe No. 30, in a little water, till the breathing and circulation are normal. If it does not yield to this treatment, and pneumonia is inevitable, adopt the treatment prescribed for that without delay, and apply it vigorously. Approaching pneumonia will be noticed by a rise in temperature. If the temperature goes above 101 ° Fahr. and the breathing continues labored, look out for pneumonia.

Prevention.—Feed a horse according to his work. If he is doing daily hard work there is very little danger of overfeeding, but if the work is light and little of it, feed sparingly on heavy grain. Give daily regular exercise. There is very much less danger of derangements if the horse goes out every day than if he only goes out once or twice a week, and he is able to do ten times the work from the fact that he is in a strong, vigorous condition—muscular without being fat.

XI. Pleurisy.

The lining of the chest and coverings of the lungs are serous membranes that secrete a serous, slippery moisture that prevents friction by rubbing of the lungs against the ribs—called the *pleura*. Inflammation of these serous membranes is known as pleurisy. It is attended with great pain, and is often followed by hydrothorax or filling of the chest with water, which is generally fatal. Pleurisy may exist alone or with pneumonia; then it is called pleuro-pneumonia.

Causes.—Any sudden exposure to cold rains; drafts in the stable, especially if the horse comes in warm. It would be very prevalent if the inflammation in these parts did not go to the feet by metastasis as often as it does. See founder or laminitis.

How to know it.—The horse has a chill, followed by high fever; great pain in the chest, shown by colicky pains; nose turned around towards the chest frequently; ears and legs are cold; breathing hurried; pulse quick, from 50 to 75 per minute; temperature raised three or four degress; elbows turned out, and a line along the lower edges of the ribs denoting a fixed position of them to prevent friction in the chest; loss of appetite; great pain evinced upon pressure with the fingers between the ribs; a grating sound heard by the ear applied to the sides, made by the rubbing of the parts internally, which are rendered dry by the inflammation.

If recovery takes place, it is usually within four days; but if it continues longer than that, effusion takes place, and the chest begins to fill with water, floating the lungs up and forming hydrothorax. If the chest does not fill more than one-third, it will usually absorb, and he will recover; but if the chest fills more than one-third full, it is usually fatal.

What to do.—If seen during the chill, put on blankets ; shelter from the cold air, and give half a teacup of whiskey in a little water, and follow it with receipe No. 40, giving a dose every two hours till he is better ; set a pail of water before him, and feed lightly. Rub the liniment, No. 41, well in to the sides, and, after six hours, repeat it. When the fever is broken, change the prescription to No. 18. When convalesence is well established, give receipe No. 22.

XII. Hydrothorax.

Causes.—This is a filling of the chest with water, following pleurisy.

How to know it.—The horse has been enduring great pain all through the attack of active inflammation, but as soon as effusion begins, and the chest begins to fill with water, the pain is relieved ; he brightens up, commences to eat, and is more comfortable, till the water floats the lungs up and interferes with the breathing. Then the countenance becomes haggard and anxious ; breathing short and fast ; breath cold, from shallow, bronchial respiration ; the extremeties are cold ; pulse very high, from 80 to 150 per minute ; tapping on the sides will produce the solid

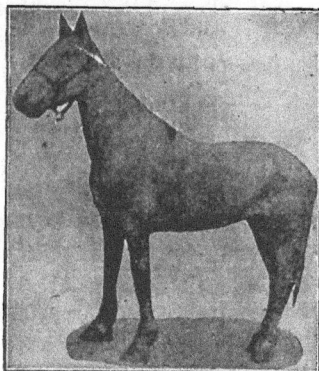

CONGESTION OF LUNGS.
Fore limbs apart and well under body. Nostrils are flapping and the eye has a deadly stare.

sound of a barrel full of water ; the ear placed to the side will fail to detect the customary respiratory murmur ; there will be lifting of the loins and elevation of the back at each effort at inspiration, that is, drawing breath in ; the ribs bulge outward ; dropsical swellings appear under the chest and belly ; the head is extended ; there is flapping of the nostrils ; regurgitation of the blood in the veins ; splashing of the water is heard in the chest when it reaches the heart ; the pulse gets smaller and smaller ; breath shorter and shorter, till he drops suffocated, as completely drowned as though he were pitched into the lake.

14

Favorable symptoms are lessening of the effusion in the chest; improvement in the breathing and pulse; return of healthy appetite, etc. But recovery is slow, and complete recovery is seldom realized, for the lung is apt to grow fast to the ribs, and stitches in the side attack him during active exercise.

What to do.—Put him in a comfortable place, dry, warm, and well-ventilated, but no drafts. Clothe warmly, and bandage the legs. If the sides have not been well blistered with receipe No. 41, apply it immediately, and repeat it every six hours, till the sides are well-blistered, and give No. 18 internally, every two hours, very persistently; if he eats nothing, drench him with oat-meal gruel. If the chest continues to fill it may be tapped, the operation being called *paracentesis thoracis*, directions for which may be found in the chapter on operations.

XIII. Chronic Cough.

Causes.—When the inflammation of the mucous membrane of either the larynx or bronchial tubes becomes chronic, the irritability of it remains and the smallest thing will produce a cough, and sometimes a fit of coughing that may last several minutes. Dust in the hay or oats, or breathed in while on the road, sudden gusts of air, pressure of the collar or throat lash, or pinching of the throat with the hand will excite the cough.

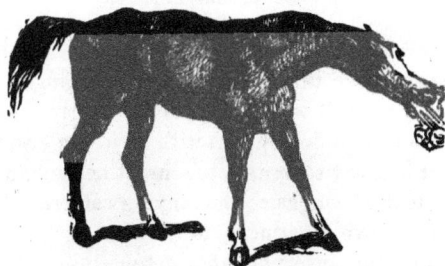

THE ACT OF COUGHING.

How to know It.—Coughs are efforts of nature to free the breathing apparatus of irritants, and they differ according to the part affected and the extent of the affection. The healthy cough is strong, full and usually followed by a sneeze to clear the nose. The throat cough is a lighter, shorter, hacking one, while that of the chest is a hollow, deep, resonant cough, except in the acute, painful stages of bronchitis, when it is almost noiseless from being so much subdued.

What to do.—Chronic cough is almost incurable when long standing, but in the more recent cases good treatment will benefit and oftentimes

15

cure. If the cough is recent, apply recipe No. 41 to the throat, well rubbed in all around and up towards the ears. Give internally the following powders :

No. 43.   1½ Ounce gum camphor,
            1 Ounce digitalis,
            2 Ounces linseed meal,
            Powder and mix.

Divide into twelve powders and give one night and morning in soft food. If one course does not cure, repeat it. If that proves ineffectual, apply blister No. 9 instead of No. 41, to the throat and give Prof. Dick's recipe as follows :

No. 44.   1 Drachm camphor,
            1 Drachm digitalis,
            1 Drachm calomel,

            Mix in a ball with syrup.

Give it as one dose ; repeat it once a day for a week, then rest a week and repeat.

If the cough is very troublesome and the appetite is poor, give the following :

No. 45.   2 Drachms diluted prussic acid,
            1 Ounce tincture of camphor,
            3 Drachms fluid extract belladona,
            1 Ounce tincture gentian.
            1 Ounce chlorate of potash,
            Water to make one pint,
            Mix.

Give one ounce three times a day, with a syringe ; open the mouth with one hand and shoot it well back into the throat. Do not attempt to hold a horse's head up to drench him with anything else than oil when he has a cough ; for it is apt to irritate the throat and might choke him.

For the treatment of coughs accompanying catarrh and laryngitis refer to them. If the above treatment fails, we would recommend the insertion of a seton under the skin of the throat and a long run at grass, if practicable. Leave the seton in three or four weeks ; wash it nice and clean once a day with hot water. Sometimes a run at grass will do more for a bad cough than all the medicine in the world.

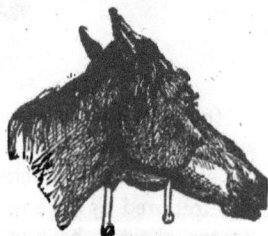

A SETON IN THE THROAT OF A HORSE.

If the cough appears to come from the chest, and pressure in the hollow just above the breast bone aggravates it, apply the blisters there, and give the same treatment otherwise as for the throat.

16

DISEASES AND ACCIDENTS OF THE ALIMENTARY CANAL.

I. Teeth—Ache, Decay, Filing--Wolf Teeth.

Causes.—Derangements of the teeth very frequently lead to grave difficulties, both local and constitutional. The teeth often become decayed, holes form in them, and tooth-ache is a common occurrence.

How to know it.—It will be detected by the horse holding his head on one side while chewing, turning his head first one way then the other,

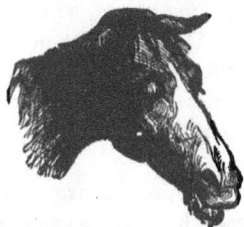

A HORSE WITH TOOTHACHE.

as if trying to remove food from a sore tooth, and doing the same when drinking, if the water is very cold. The disease often extends up the tooth, or starts in the form of ulceration on the fang, and breaks out into the nose, causing a discharge from the nostril on the side on which the rotten tooth is located. A chronic discharge from a tooth is often mistaken for nasal gleet, and sometimes for glanders, on account of the disagreeable odor, which will be recognized as that characteristic of diseased bone.

Sometimes the ulceration, when of a lower tooth, breaks out at the angle of the lower jaw, and sometimes extends to the root of the tongue and to all the soft tissues between the branches of the lower jaw ; in one instance that came under the notice of the writer, the disease proved fatal to a valuable horse.

The teeth frequently get broken by chewing on stones taken up with oats, and when one molar tooth gets broken off, the opposite tooth, not having anything to wear against, gets very long and sticks into the opposite gum, and makes mastication very painful. The edges of the molar teeth get sharp from the fact that they wear bevelling—the edges must necessarily sharpen as they wear ; the upper rows bevel downwards and outwards, the edges cutting the cheeks, and the lower rows bevel upwards and inwards, cutting the tongue.

The broken and sharp teeth make mastication not only painful, but almost impossible, consequently the horse bolts the food half chewed, which causes indigestion, colic, dyspepsia, hidebound, emaciation, etc., any of which may run on to a fatal termination. The food is frequently quidded and dropped into the manger.

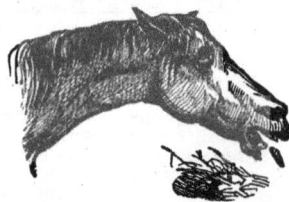

Colts, when shedding their teeth, often suffer a great deal from sore mouths, which

A HORSE QUIDDING.

causes them to look rough and scaly until the old teeth are shed, and new ones grow.

What to do.—In case of a discharge from the nose, always examine the teeth, and if any are decayed so as to cause the trouble, remove them. If a tooth extends below the others on account of the opposite one being broken, file it off even with the others. If the edges get sharp, so as to scarify the cheeks and tongue, file them off round. There are files made expressly for that purpose. The edges only need filing; the surfaces get very rough, but that is intended to be so by nature; it is her millstone to grind the grain; and the arrangement of the tooth material is such that the more it wears the sharper it gets.

In case of a parrot mouth, where the upper incisors project over the lower ones, the horse is unable to graze, and the mouth, as far as age is concerned, presents a horrible appearance, passing for double the age he really is. Either file or saw them off even with the lower row.

Wolf Teeth.—These are small, insignificant teeth, that come immediately in front of the upper rows of molars. It is a popular idea that these affect the nerve running to the eye and cause moon-blindness, weak eyes, etc. But

PARROT MOUTH.

it is a whim; they do no possible harm, except, perhaps, to wound the cheek by its being pulled against the wolf tooth by the bit. But they do no possible good, and, consequently are just as well, and a little better, out. Take a pair of blacksmith's pinchers and pull them out. They are usually only in the gums, and come out easily. When the new teeth of colts come before the old ones are out, the old ones should be removed, to make room for the new.

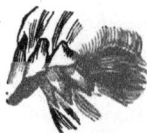

II. Tongue Laceration.

Causes.—The tongue is sometimes bitten by falling and striking on the mouth; torn with the halter chain, or by being pulled forcibly out of the mouth on one side, being cut against the sharp molar teeth.

18

What to do.—Wounds on the tongue heal readily. If the end is torn half-way off, or less, it will heal, but will not grow together, but may be left, and no inconvenience will be felt; but if it is more than half torn off, it will be found advisable to cut it clear off. Dress wounds of the tongue with the following lotion:

_ No. 46.   1 Ounce borax,
            1 Ounce honey,
            1 Pint water,
            Mix.

Dry the sore with a sponge, and rub on the lotion three times a day.

Sometimes it is necessary to amputate the tongue, on account of wounds and accidents. It is quite feasible, but requires the skill of a qualified veterinary surgeon.

III. Sore Mouth.

Causes.—The mouth is often made sore by the bit, by caustic substances in the food and medicine, by too hot mashes, etc. The bit often

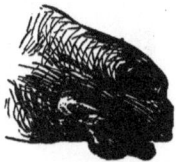

SORE MOUTH.

With the angles excoriated by the bit.

excoriates the angles of the mouth, and, if allowed to continue doing harm, the mouth soon becomes caloused, and loses all sensibility. Sometimes the bit injures the lower jaw bone so as to kill a portion of it, when it will become a foreign substance and slough out, leaving a very sore mouth.

This is most often seen in violent

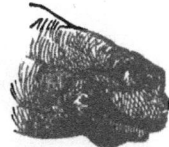

SORE MOUTH.

With the angles and cheeks swollen, caloused and insensitive.

pullers and when the curb bit is used. The oval portion of a curb bit often presses upon the roof of the mouth and does a great amount of injury.

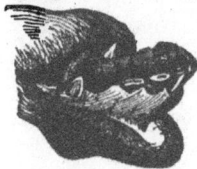

INJURY BY THE BIT.

A mouth with the bone badly injured by the bit, the left side being much swollen around the tusk.

How to know it.—When any portion of the mouth is swollen and sore, examine it carefully and locate the cause if possible. When the bones or roof of the mouth are injured, there will be great soreness and some swelling.

What to do.—Remove the cause, that is, leave the bit out of the mouth for several days. If

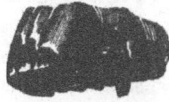

MISUSE OF CURB.

The roof of the mouth injured by the curved part of the curb bit.

the angles of the mouth are raw, apply recipe No. 32 three times a day. If the bones are injured and exposed apply No. 39 three times a day;

if the flesh is not broken it would be advisable to scarify it to allow it to break through the tough skin more easily, and examine it carefully each day to see when the dead piece of bone is loose, and remove it. Then dress the wound with the same lotion, (No 39) till the bone is covered by healthy granulations, then dress it with No. 46. Do not use the bit in such a mouth under two months at least.

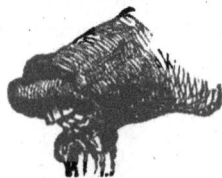

SCALDED MOUTH.

From giving strong caustic medicine pure.

When the mouth is scalded by giving strong medicine, pure, instead of diluting it as directed on the label, the whole inside of the mouth will be found to be swollen, red, and if very bad, will skin in spots. Swab it out with recipe No. 46 three times a day.

IV. Lampas.

This is an imaginary disease. It is supposed by most people that when a horse does not eat he must have the lampas, and they proceed to

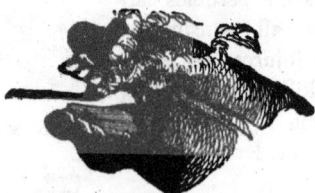

BURNING FOR LAMPAS.

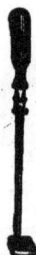

LAMPAS IRON.

The old time instrument of torture.

burn out one or two of the bars in the roof of the mouth which are placed there by nature to prevent the food dribbling from the mouth, which it would do were it not for these bars in the roof of the mouth. They all point or turn backwards towards the throat, and have a tendency to work the food back. It is the same in the human mouth.

Sometimes the one or two bars nearest the incisors become inflamed, especially with colts when teething.

What to do.—If the bars are red instead of a bright flesh color, and extend below the teeth, take a pen knife and scarify them gently; this will be sufficient. Never countenance the burning nor any other barbarous practice.

V. Pharyngitis.

That portion of the æsophagas or gullet that lies in the throat, above the larynx is called the pharynx. Inflammation of it is pharyngitis.

Causes.—It is usually caused by some foreign substance lodging there or by extension to the pharynx of inflammation from the larynx and nasal chambers. It is usually associated with pharyngitis and catarrh, strangles, quinsy, etc.

How to know it.—Painful swallowing, and sometimes a total inability to swallow is seen; the water returns by the nose while drinking, and the food is quidded. More, or less enlargement of the throat and glands on the outside, tenderness upon pressure, and the neck straightened and the head extended, will be the symptoms usually noticed.

What to do.—If any foreign substance is suspected, examine the throat and remove anything that may be found. Apply a counter irritant in the form of the recipe No. 41. Give internally, mixture No. 21. Feed on soft feed, such as scalded oats, boiled barley, bran mashes, etc. If it continues longer than a week, give oat meal gruel injections—two quarts every four or five hours. Cook the gruel the same as for the table.

VI. Choking.

Causes.—Horses very seldom get choked; but in some instances they bolt their food, especially when fed on dry ground feed, and swallow it before it is properly moistened with saliva, and it accumulates in the gullet sometimes as large as your double fist, usually about six or eight inches from the throat. It often gives rise to a great amount of flatulence. Sometimes it leaves a sac in the gullet, from the distension of the fibres of its walls; the sac is called *dilatation* of the *œsophagus*.

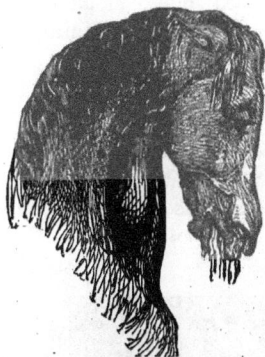

What to do.—Give the horse a couple of swallows of raw lindseed oil, and manipulate the lump, and try and pass it on a little at a time, till it is all worked down; if this proves ineffectual, the probang must be used, but

CHOKING.

A horse trying to raise the food stuck in the throat from a stricture in the gullet.

great care and caution are necessary not to keep it in too long, and not to push it through the walls of the gullet. A horse cannot breathe with the probang in his throat, therefore it is dangerous to leave it in longer than one minute at a time. If the obstruction is near enough to the throat, so it can be reached with the hand, run your arm down and remove it. As a last resort, when all other means have been exhausted, cut down upon the substance and remove it. Make the opening in the skin large enough to get a hand in, but make the hole in the gullet as small as possible,

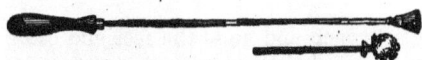

TWO FORMS OF PROBANG

The probang with a piece of sponge on the end is far the best.

just large enough to get one finger in, and break down the obstruction.

21

Cut carefully so as not to wound the jugular vein. Draw the edges of the gullet together with either catgut or silk, and dress it twice a day with lotion No. 39. Sew the skin with silk, and after dressing the wound with the above lotion, saturate a wad of oakum with the lotion and tie it over the wound. Keep the horse on very sloppy food, and very little of it,

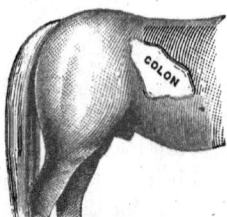

WHERE TO TAP FOR STOMACH STAGGERS.

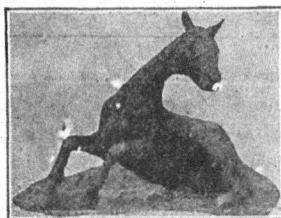

CEREBRO SPINAL MENINGITIS.
Horse is Delirious and Partially Paralyzed.

mostly oatmeal gruel, until the wound in the gullet is healed. Avoid making the opening if possible, for it is very hard indeed at all times, and sometimes utterly impossible, to make it heal, and a fatal termination is often the result.

VII. Gastritis.

Causes.—This is inflammation of the stomach, caused by over-eating at any one time, getting into a clover field or at an oat bin or corn crib. Eating poisonous herbs or accidentally eating poison also causes it. The

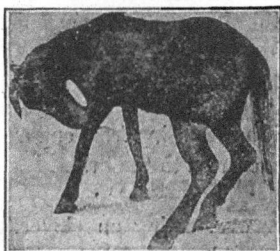

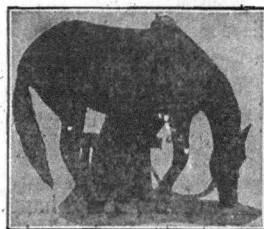

MOVEMENTS IN INFLAMMATION OF THE BOWELS.
Horse gets up and down slowly and hesitatingly. Often mistaken for colic.

disease has a tendency to leave the stomach and go to the feet and cause founder. On account of this tendency we seldom have occasion to treat gastritis.

22

How to know It.—There is a tendency to wind colic, the food not being digested rapidly enough, decomposition sets in and leads to flatulence. There is usually a loss of appetite, and sometimes symptoms of nausea, such as turning up the nose.

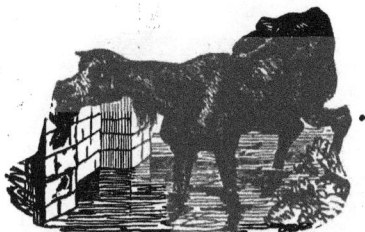

CHRONIC GASTRITIS.

A horse quenching the excessive thirst of chronic gastritis.

What to do.—Give a complete change of food; if corn and oats have been fed, change to bran, carrots and boiled barley, and if in season; give green food. Give raw linseed oil in half pint doses once a day till the bowels are quite soft, and feed a little oil-cake meal, a pint once a day. If wind accumulates after eating, give the following as a drench :

No. 47.   1 Teaspoonful bicarbonate of soda,
            1 Ounce extract of ginger,
            ½ Pint water,
              Mix and give as one dose.

If thirst is excessive, give half an ounce of chlorate in the water, well dissolved, twice a day. This excessive thirst is often seen as a symptom of the disease when it has become chronic.

VIII. Stomach Staggers.

This is a sleepy, dumpish, stupid condition resulting from engorgement, and through the nerves the impression is carried to the brain, and stupor is the effect.

Causes.—It frequently happens after over-eating on clover, or the horse gets into the garden and fills up on cabbages or roots of any kind.

How to know It.—The horse is usually found standing in a stupid manner as though asleep, perfectly quiet, and perhaps with his mouth full of food ; he is oblivious to all around ; place one foot across the other, and he will leave it so ; prick him and he may wake up for an instant, but subsides again as quickly.

23

What to do.—Put him in a safe place : remove all food ; give him very little water, and give a dose of purgative medicine as follows :

No. 48.   6 Drachms barbadoes aloes,
                 1 Pint raw linseed oil,
                 Mix.

Give as one dose. As soon as he is sufficiently recovered give him walking exercise. If the purgative does not work in the course of twenty-

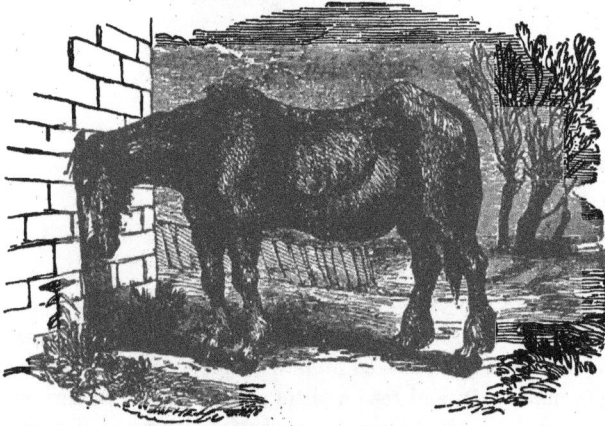

A HORSE WITH STOMACH OR SLEEPY STAGGERS.

four hours, give injections of warm water and soft soap every hour till purgation is obtained.

Prevention.—Avoid engorgement ; feed on bulky food.

IX. Dyspepsia.

Causes.—This is rather uncommon, but is occasionally seen in horses that have been fed artificially for any great length of time, especially if highly fed.

How to know it.—There will be a general unthrifty appearance to the horse ; he will be thin ; coat rough and staring, hide bound ; and the surest symptom of all is the yellowish color and offensive smell of the manure. After a while the appetite wanes ; he gets hungry, and will rush at the food as though he would swallow the whole at once, eats a few mouthfuls and leaves the rest ; perhaps he will nibble a little more, but will not eat as though he relished it. He gradually grows worse, till he becomes a mere skeleton.

What to do.—If practicable, give him three or four months at grass ; first examine the teeth, and remedy any defect. If it is not the right time of year to turn out to grass, give a complete change of food · carrots, turnips, apples, boiled barley, scalded oats, and bran mashes. Feed no corn at all. Give a dose of purgative medicine, recipe No. 28. When the purgation is all over, give the tonic No. 34, in soft feed. If the appetite is poor, so that he won't eat the powder, give No. 35. Continue it a week, then stop a week, and repeat.

X. Spasmodic Colic.

The term colic, means pain in the colon, (one of the large intestines), but is accepted as the name for all pain in the abdomen. It is often called belly-ache. It is always very serious, indeed, for two reasons—it is terribly painful, and is very apt to run into inflammation of the bowels, which is usually fatal.

Spasmodic colic is pain in the bowels, from the violent, spasmodic contraction and cramp of the muscular coat of the bowels. It is called spasmodic on account of the pain and cramps being spasmodic and not contin-

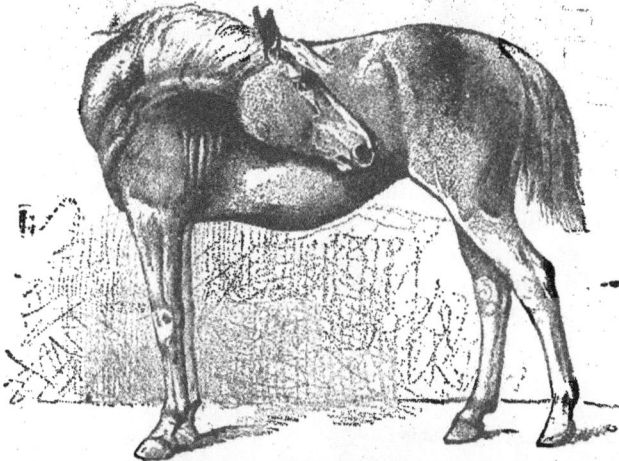

FIRST STAGE OF SPASMODIC COLIC

uous; there are moments of relief from the pain, in which the animal will be quite at his ease, but it is apt to come on again after a few moments.

Some horses are particularly subject to colic, owing to a ravenous manner of eating and drinking, consequently they have it from time to time, and usually die with it after a few repetitions.

Causes.—It is caused by some irritant in the bowels—indigestible matter; also by large draughts of cold water, particularly if the horse is warm. Colicky pains are very often symptoms of other diseases.

How to know it.—In the first stage, the horse will begin to be uneasy; looks around; raises up his hind feet towards his belly; steps around from one side of the stall to the other; stops eating; will curl as if to lie down

In the second stage, he lies down and gets up again after lying, perhaps, a couple of minutes; in the third stage, he rolls, kicks, sweats profusely, has a haggard countenance, is inclined to turn upon his back, and remains so. In mild cases, after kicking for half an hour or so, the

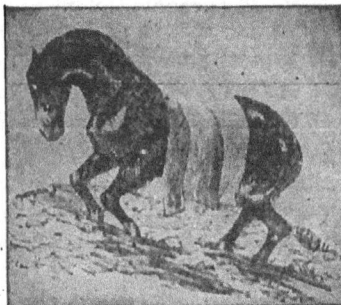

SECOND STAGE OF SPASMODIC COLIC.

horse usually gets better, the pain all passes off, and he returns to his accustomed spirits and habits; but if it does not go off in the course of half an hour, and from that to two or three hours, it is apt to run into enteritis, and kill him.

What to do.—Give mild, diffusible stimulants, as early and quickly as possible. Give either of the following:

No. 49.
  2 Ounce whiskey,
  1 Ounces extract of ginger,
  ½ Pint water,
    Mix.

Give as one dose. Or this:

No. 50.
  Sweet spirits of nitre, 1½ oz.
  Fluid extract of ginger, ½ oz.
  Water to make ½ pint.
    Mix.

Give as one dose. Always, when possible, give warm water injections with a very little soap in it, just to make it a little slippery. Give the horse a soft, roomy place to roll in, and if he has the colic at all bad, give a couple of days rest afterwards, feeding on soft food. Give the abdomen friction, and put on a blanket to avoid his cooling off too soon.

When the worst part of the pain is over, a little walking exercise will be beneficial. If after giving the first dose the pain continues more than half an hour, repeat it every half hour till relief is obtained; but if it does not yield with three or four doses, give the following:

No. 51.   1 Quart raw linseed oil,
           ½ Ounce chloroform,
                  Mix

Give as one dose. In half an hour, if the pain is continuous, **give**

No. 52.   Chloral hydrate, ½ oz.
           Water, ½ pint.
           Mix, dissolve and give immediately.

Give as one dose with a syringe. Repeat it every half hour if necessary to keep him quiet. If this does not effect a cure, refer to treatment for enteritis, for it certainly has run into inflammation of the bowels.

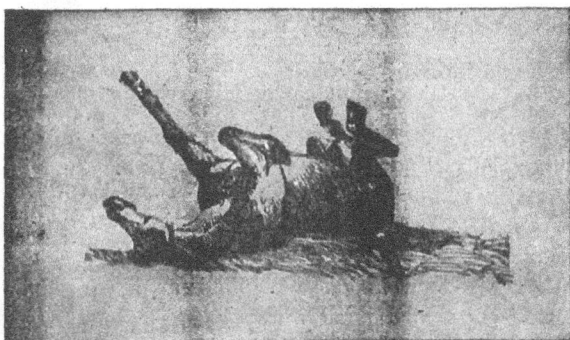

THIRD STAGE OF SPASMODIC COLIC.

XI. Flatulent Colic.

Causes.—The nature of this disease is· acute indigestion. Either weak digestion, or a suspension of digestion entirely, allows the undigested food to decompose, and while undergoing that process, fermentation sets up, gas is evolved, and the horse bloats up, sometimes to an alarming extent, even to cause death by suffocation or rupture of the stomach, intestines or diaphragm. It is most common where corn is fed freely, and is apt to come on when the horse is taken out to work or drive immediately after eating. The active exercise retards or wholly interrupts digestion, and the moment digestion stops, decomposition sets in and the evolution of gas begins. It is very weakening and often fatal. It usually lasts about two to four hours, but sometimes lingers for ten or twelve, and sometimes proves fatal in half or three-quarters of an hour.

How to know it.—The characteristic symptom is the bloating with gas, and there is always a great amount of pain. The horse rolls, kicks, paws, tries to lie on his back, gets up and down, sweats tremendously, has a haggard look in his face, gulps wind and food from the stomach in small quantities through his nose; and the food thus discharged is usually green and very sour. The nostrils are distended, breathing rapid and breath cold from the shallow breathing; the pulse is quickened at the start, but gradually grows harder and smaller as the fatal termination approaches; the belly becomes so distended that the flanks are above the points of the hips; and in some cases, when lying down, the legs are so spread from the distension of the belly that the animal is unable to get up. If it lasts very long, the nervous system becomes exhausted; the

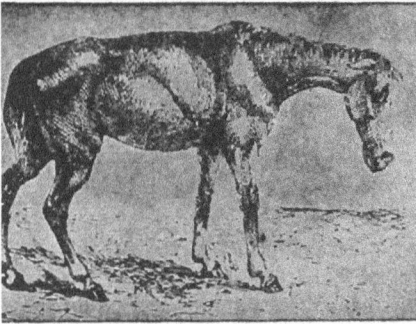

FLATULANT COLIC—FIRST STAGE.

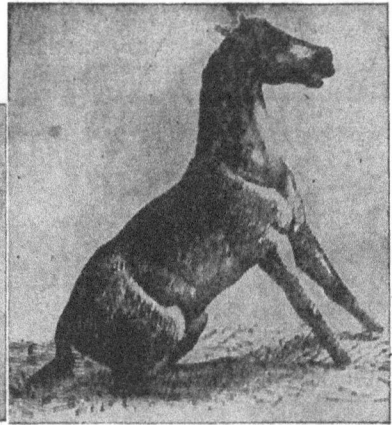

FLATULENT COLIC, RUPTURED OR LAST STAGE.

muscles around the chest, shoulders and neck cramp and draw down so as to almost pull the horse to the ground, and he will sometimes scream out like a child from the pain. The ears and extremities get deathly cold.

If rupture takes place, he will sit on his haunches like a dog, turn up his upper lip as though nauseated and try to vomit; but owing to the peculiar formation of the stomach the horse cannot vomit. The pulse gets weaker and smaller till he falls and dies from nervous exhaustion. When he dies in earlier stages, it is from suffocation; the distension of the stomach and bowels presses on the lungs so hard that it forces them up into so small a compass that they cannot work, and suffocation is the result.

Favorable symptoms are cessation of pain ; free evacuation of gas per rectum ; pulse returns to its normal condition ; ears and extremities regain their natural temperature ; sweating stops, and the horse returns to his feed and customary habits.

What to do.—As soon as it is discovered, give the following :

No. 53.   1 Tablespoonful bicarbonate soda (saleratus),
            1 Teacupful water,
            Mix.

Give as one dose, and repeat it, if necessary, in ten minutes.

Give warm water injections, being careful not to push the nozzle of the syringe through a gut ; for the intestines crowd backward so hard that it is very difficult to give injection enough to amount to anything, although it is best to try.   If the soda does no good, give the following :

No. 54.   Oil of turpentine, 1 oz.
            Raw linseed oil, 7 ounces.
            Mix

Give as one dose, and repeat it in **fifteen minutes, if necessary.**   It this proves ineffectual, give

No. 55.   1 Ounce chloroform,
            1 Pint raw linseed oil,
            Mix.

Give as one dose, and repeat. if necessary, **in half an hour.**

Bind hot water rags to the belly, and keep them hot.

As a last resort, if the flatulence does not yield to the above treatment, the trocar and cannula may be used.   Let it be a small one, not over one quarter inch in diameter and three inches long ; find the center of a triangle formed by the last rib, point of the hip, and the edges nearest the flank of the spines in the loins ; clip off the hair, and pass the trochar in slowly

TROCHAR PROVIDED WITH
CANNULA FOR PUNCTUR-
ING THE ABDOMEN.

and firmly, pointing it in and down at the same time, so as to avoid wounding the kidney ; leave the cannula in there, but draw out the trocar, and, if the gut that is distended is tapped, the gas will rush out. Sometimes fœcal matter will clog the cannula ; if so, pass in a small piece of whalebone, or other probe, to remove it from the lower end. If no gut is tapped, try the same operation on the other side.   It makes no difference which side is tapped, for there is no paunch adherent to the side of horses, as in cattle.   The treatment by the mouth may be kept up while this is done.

When they drop from suffocation, or when ruprure takes place, it is too late to do anything ; but, in every case, persevere till either one or the other of these tells you further effort is useless.

XII. Rupture of the Stomach, Intestines or Diaphragm.

Causes.—This occurs in violent cases of flatulence. When the generation of gas is excessive in the stomach or the intestines, they are liable to rupture, and let the food out into the abdominal cavity, or from the

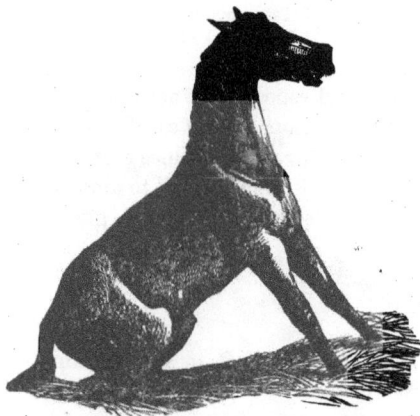

UNNATURAL ATTITUDE INDICATIVE OF ABDOMINAL INJURY.

tremendous pressure against the diaphragm, it is liable to rupture and let the intestines into the chest among the lungs and heart. Either case is fatal, the animal dying from shock to the nervous system, hemorrhage and suffocation.

How to know it.—The horse will sit on his haunches; but this is not a characteristic symptom of itself, for we see it occasionally in spasmodic colic, and often in enteritis; the horse will turn up his nose with an intensely disgusted expression on his countenance, but this, too, is often seen in colic and enteritis; he will try to vomit, which is a characteristic symptom, and the muscles and legs will tremble and shake as if with cold; the ears and legs get cold; cold sweat breaks out in patches; the mouth

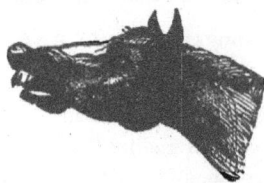

NOSE STRAINED UPWARD.

gets cold, the pulse grows smaller and smaller, till it becomes imperceptible, and death claims the patient in the course of half an hour to two hours.

XIII. Constipation.

When the fœcal matter in the intestines gets dry and hard, and resists the peristaltic effort of the bowels to pass it on, or when there is no peristaltic motion to the bowel, and the food lies quiet in one spot, there is an obstruction to all intents and purposes, which is called constipation, or costiveness.

Causes.—When the food dries and hardens so that it cannot be passed on, it is due to an insufficient quantity of water in the bowel, owing to its all going to the kidneys, or it is due to the horse not drinking enough, or to inactivity of the liver and other glands that supply the bowels with juices. When it is from a want of peristaltic motion, it is due to nervous weakness in the bowels.

How to know it.—Little or no fœtal matter is passed; what is passed is hard and dry; mild colicky pains are felt at intervals of half an hour or so. The horse may continue to eat and otherwise appear all right, but as it runs on, the pains will come oftener and be more acute till it runs into enteritis.

What to do.—If the pulse is natural and the colicky pains slight and far between, give recipe No. 23; also give warm water and soap injections. If the pains continue and increase, give a quart of raw oil and recipe No. 52. If it does not yield to this, give the following:

No. 56. 1 Quart raw oil,
 1 Ounce tincture nux vomica,
 Mix.

Give as one dose. Repeat recipe No. 52 often enough to keep down the pain. If the pain seems to be increasing and the constipation obstinate, apply to the belly, well rubbed in, the following:

No. 57. 1 Ounce croton oil,
 3 Ounces raw linseed oil,
 Mix.

Repeat recipe No. 56 every six hours till a passage is effected. Repeat the injections once an hour, but put in less soap each time. If it is necessary to repeat them more than four or five times, use clear water without soap.

XIV. Diarrhœa and Superpurgation.

These are watery evacuations from the bowels, and are the opposite to constipation.

Causes.—In diarrhœa there is an excessive secretion of the juices of the system, owing usually to some irritant in the bowels, but sometimes to too laxative food. Superpurgation is due to an overdose of purgative medicine.

How to know it.—The evacuations are frequent and watery; after running a while the bowels become irritable and the patient strains a good deal and becomes weak; the pulse gets feeble; the mouth clammy; the ears and extremities cold; the eyes and nose pale; the horse grinds his teeth, and refuses food; thirst is excessive. The temperature of the body taken with the thermometer is down, perhaps to 95 ° Fahr. If it goes down to 93 °, the disease is almost sure to terminate fatally.

What to do.—If it is a straight case of diarrhœa—that is, without any purgative having been given—give a complete change of food and the following:

No. 58.
1 Ounce prepared chalk,
½ Ounce fluid extract of ginger,
1 Drachm Salol,
½ Pint starch gruel,
Mix.

Give as one dose, and repeat it, if necessary, after three or four hours. Give him water with flour stirred in to drink, but restrict the quantity to about two quarts every three or four hours. If this does not stop it after giving two or three doses of the medicine, give the following:

No, 59.
½ Pint raw linseed oil,
1 Ounce tincture catechu,
Mix.

Give as one dose. If superpurgation is the trouble, give the flour and water to drink. If this does not check it in five or six hours, give in addition:

No. 60.
1 Ounce tincture catechu,
½ Ounce tincture camphor,
1 Drachm Salol,
1 Pint starch gruel,
Mix.

Give as one dose. Repeat it if necessary every four hours. Restrict the drinking a little, and feed lightly when the appetite returns.

XV. Dysentery.

The nature of this disease is bloody evacuations with great straining, There is inflammation of the mucous membrane of the large intestines, with more or less fever and great irritability of the intestinal tract.

Causes.—Neglected diarrhœa and superpurgation; too acid a condition of the bowels; impure, indigestible and musty food; and foul atmosphere.

How to know it.—By the bloody evacuations; severe, frequent and ineffectual attempts to pass fœcal matter; colicky pains; considerable fever; great thirst; no appetite; pulse quick, weak and compressible. It is rather rare in the horse; when it does exist, worms are often found, too, and are thought by some to assist in the cause of it.

What to do. Give recipe No. 59, and give injections of starch with one ounce of laudanum in each injection; repeat the latter every half

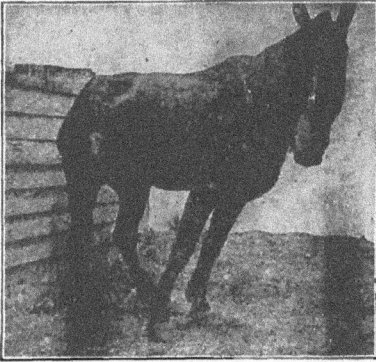

IMPACTION OF LARGE BOWEL.

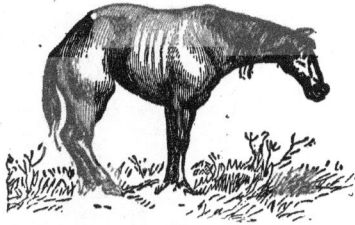

A SUFFERER FROM CONSTIPATION.
The tucked-up belly, the attitude, and general expression of suffering are plainly shown.

hour. In one hour after taking No. 59 give No. 58, and in another hour, if the straining continues, give No. 60, and the following injection:

No. 61.
> 1 Ounce sulphuric ether,
> 1 Pint starch gruel,
> Mix.

If no improvement takes place in the course of ten hours, give a pint of raw oil and repeat the injection every half hour.

XVI. Enteritis.

Inflammation of the bowels takes two forms, according to the part affected. Enteritis is inflammation of the mucous lining of the bowel; the next subject, peritonitis, is inflammation of the outer or serous covering of the bowel.

Causes.—Irritating substances in the food; catching cold which settles in the bowels, continuation of colic, either spasmodic or flatulent; and poison.

How to know It.—There is continuous pain, light at first, and increasing as the inflammation develops. It is different from colic, for which it might be taken by an ordinary observer, in that it is continuous, while colic is intermittent; in colic, the horse throws himself down; in enteritis he lies down carefully; the pulse is raised to seventy-five or eighty, or even a hundred

33

beats to the minute ; the countenance wears an anxious look ; he is very uneasy ; when not getting up and down he is turning around ; if in a box stall, he looks around to his sides, paws, raises his legs up towards the body ; the breathing is hurried ; there is profuse sweating ; the pulse is soft at first, but grows gradually harder, faster, and at last it gets wiry, and finally imperceptible ; the extremities get cold, and the horse wears himself out

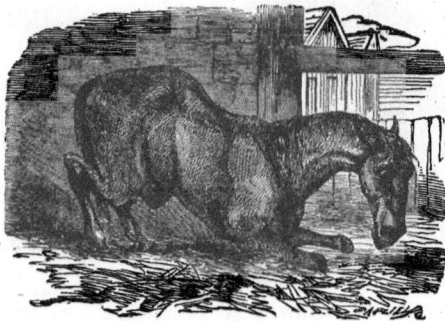

POSITION ASSUMED BY HORSE SUFFERING FROM ABDOMINAL INJURY.

with the pain and constant moving about. Towards the last, the pain will apparently abate a little ; he will stand quiet for a while ; brace his legs till he cannot resist any longer, and will reel and drop, the hind end first, generally. He dies in the course of eight to twenty hours after the first symptom, but in some instances the horse will die in six hours after the very first symptom. Sometimes they get perfectly crazy with the pain, and they will rear, run, climb over anything, tear down the stalls, etc. They can bear no pressure on the belly without pain.

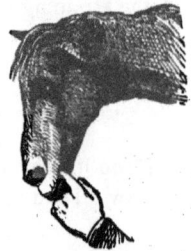

ENTERITIS.

A test for enteritis, the mouth usually being found hot and dry.

What to do.—Treatment is of very little use, for a genuine case of enteritis is always incurable, but it is best to try always. At first, it is usually taken for colic, and the prescribed drenches are given for that disease ; but when you notice the pain is continuous and the pulse runs up, it is sufficient evidence to locate the trouble as inflammation of the lining of the large intestines ; then give No. 56, and apply a mustard paste to the belly. After it has been on an hour, wash it off and repeat it, or apply No. 41, and confine the fumes with a blanket. A few minutes after giving the oil, give No. 52 ; repeat the latter every half hour, if necessary to keep him easy. Give No. 30, continuously, in addition to the others. Also give injections of soap and water. If the pulse continues to quicken and get hard, repeat the oil every two or three hours, and apply No. 57 to the belly where the mus-

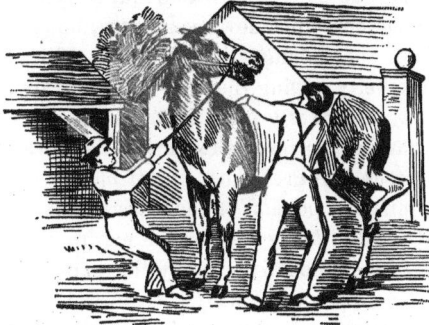

ANOTHER TEST FOR ENTERITIS.

A horse manifesting tenderness upon pressure on the belly in enteritis.

tard was. If the oil works through, there is a chance of success; then just let the horse remain perfectly quiet for several days, give oat-meal gruel to drink.

Post mortem examination shows the bowel affected to be almost black from congestion, inflammation, and mortification. The dis

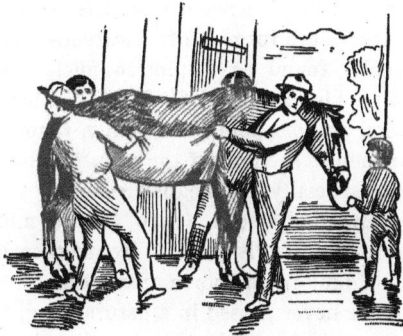

APPLICATION OF AN AMMONIACAL BLISTER.

confines itself to about a yard of the gut. The tissue of the intestine will be swollen sometimes over an inch thick.

XVII. Peritonitis.

This is inflammation of the outer covering of the bowel; it is less rapid in its course, and less painful. It may last a week or so, or it may kill in ten or twelve hours.

Causes.—Wounds in the abdominal cavity, exposure to cold storms, kicks in the belly, etc.

How to know it.—The pulse is quick—from sixty to seventy-five, and is hard and wiry; the horse lies down very easy, but gets up quick; loss of appetite. When the inflammation does not kill, effusion of water takes place into the belly, giving the horse the appearance of dropsy by the large abdomen. There is great pain upon pressure on the abdomen.

Post mortem examination reveals extensive discoloration of the bowels and surrounding tissue. A great quantity of bloody matter is floating in the cavity. The inflamed portion of the intestines is very much swollen.

What to do.—Give No. 56 as soon as the nature of the disease is recognized. Give No. 52 occasionally to allay the pain, and apply No. 57 to the belly. Give No. 30. continuously for several doses, till the pulse is improved. In case the abdomen fills with water, it may be tapped by passing in the trocar and cannula—the smallest size—through the centre of the belly, and through the hard, fibrous band running down the center. It is called *paracentesis abdomenis*, and should be performed by experts only.

XVIII. Calculi.

Intestinal calculi are not very common, although they are occasionally met with. It is very probable, that if all the cases of death from bowel troubles were examined *post mortem*, calculi would be quite often found, as that is the only way their presence can be determined.

Causes.—These stones are formed of calcareous material laid on in layers, and are usually found enveloping a nucleus of some kind—a piece of a nail, or a pebble, or a wad of hair, etc. They sometimes attain to enormous sizes and weight, and are usually round or oval. These stones are most common in sections of the country where hard well water is used for drinking, especially in lime districts.

Dust balls are common in horses that are fed on mill-sweepings; the dust accumulates around oat hulls or chaff from other grain. As many as a dozen have been found in one horse after death.

Calculi are seldom or never passed in a natural way, but make sacks in the bowel, and lie there till by accident they are dislodged and roll out into the passage, and form an obstruction, cause a stoppage, inflammation and death.

How to know it.—In addition to the symptoms of enteritis, the patient will frequently sit on his haunches like a dog. This is not a characteristic symptom, but in cases where calculi have been found, it was a prominent symptom.

What to do.—Nothing more can be done than to treat the symptoms, which are those of enteritis. Back raking is advisable, but it is not among the probabilities that the stones would be near enough to the rectum, to be reached by the hand.

XIX. Intussusception and Gut Tie.

This is the slipping of a part of a gut into another part, like turning a finger of a glove partly wrong side out. It is rather uncommon. A case was lately seen by the writer, in which the blind end of the *cœcum* was turned into the other part, the fold coming at the intersection of the small intestines.

Causes.—The cause of intussusception is purely accidental.

How to know it.—There are signs of bowel trouble ; colicky pains that come on gradually ; the horse looks around ; paws ; stretches at full length, which is a tolerably characteristic symptom ; gets up and down ; the pulse rises and has a tendency to become hard and wiry ; legs and ears get cold ; patches of cold sweat break out over the body ; the pulse gets smaller and harder ; the muscles tremble, and death soon follows, which is caused by strangulation of the gut and mortification of the part affected.

Post mortem examination shows great swelling of the gut, sometimes to an inch thick, and the mortified portion will be black.

What to do.—As soon as any rise or change in the pulse is detected, especially if there is stretching and colicky pains, give recipe No. 56, hot water injections, and hot water rugs to the belly. If this does not give relief in an hour, give No. 55, and repeat it every two hours till relief is got ; in between these doses, if necessary to keep down the pain, give No. 52. In some cases the intestines will return to their proper place, and their functions go on naturally again, but in some cases all efforts are unavailing, and death takes place in from ten to thirty hours.

Gut Tie.—This is similar in effect ; the bowel gets into a half knot and strangulation follows the same as in intussusception.

Gut Twist.—This is a twisting of a gut by turning partly over. If it does not right itself, strangulation and death are the inevitable result.